The Taste of Portugal:

A
Food Lover's Guide to the
Best of Portuguese Dishes &
Wines

Wanda Welch

Table of Contents

Introduction

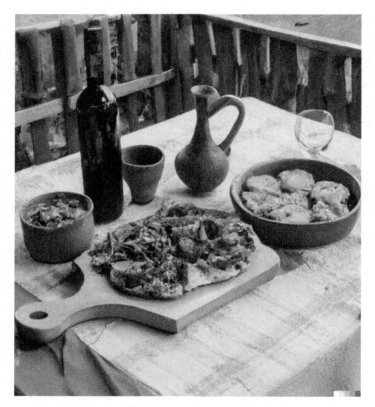

Welcome to "The Taste of Portugal: A Food Lover's Guide to the Best Dishes and Wines". This guide book is for those who are looking to explore the rich and diverse culinary traditions of Portugal.

Portuguese cuisine is a unique blend of Mediterranean and Atlantic influences, featuring an abundance of fresh seafood, hearty meats, and flavorful spices. From the famous Bacalhau (salt cod) to the sweet and creamy Pasteis de Nata (custard tarts), Portugal offers a wide variety of dishes that will tantalize your taste buds.

The aim of this guide book is to provide you with a comprehensive overview of the best dishes and wines that Portugal has to offer. Whether you're a seasoned foodie or a curious traveler, this guide will help you navigate the culinary landscape of this beautiful country.

In this guide, we'll explore the traditional dishes that have been enjoyed by generations of Portuguese families, as well as newer culinary trends that have emerged in recent years. We'll also take a look at the various regional specialties that can be found throughout Portugal, from the seafood-heavy cuisine of the coast to the hearty stews of the interior.

But our guide doesn't stop at just food. We'll also introduce you to some of the best Portuguese wines, including the famous port wine from the Douro Valley, as well as other lesser-known but equally delicious varieties.

To make this guide as user-friendly as possible, we've organized it into different sections based on type of dish or wine. Each section provides a brief overview of the dish or wine, its history, and its cultural significance in Portugal. We've also included a list of recommended restaurants and wineries where you can try these dishes and wines for yourself.

In addition to providing information about the food and wine itself, we'll also offer practical tips for ordering and enjoying them in Portugal. This includes advice on etiquette, as well as suggestions for pairing dishes with wines and other beverages.

One of the key goals of this guide is to make the culinary traditions of Portugal accessible to everyone. While some dishes and wines may seem intimidating at first, we've provided easy-to-understand explanations and frameworks to help you appreciate their flavors and significance.

We believe that food is one of the most important ways to experience a new culture, and we hope that this guide will help you do just that. Whether you're traveling to

Portugal or simply looking to expand your culinary horizons at home, we're confident that this guide will provide you with the knowledge and inspiration you need to discover the best that Portuguese cuisine has to offer.

In conclusion, "The Taste of Portugal: A Food Lover's Guide to the Best Dishes and Wines" is a comprehensive guide to the rich culinary traditions of Portugal. We hope that it will inspire you to explore the diverse and delicious flavors of this beautiful country and to appreciate the cultural significance of its food and wine. So sit back, relax, and enjoy the journey!

Chapter 1: The Essence of Portuguese Cuisine

Portuguese cuisine is a rich and diverse culinary tradition that has been shaped by centuries of history, geography, and culture. From the fresh seafood of the coast to the hearty stews of the interior, Portuguese cuisine offers a wide variety of flavors and textures that reflect the country's unique culinary heritage.

In this chapter, we'll explore the history and characteristics of Portuguese cuisine, as well as the key ingredients that are essential to its distinct flavor profile.

A Brief History of Portuguese Cuisine

Portuguese cuisine has its roots in the country's long and storied history. From the Roman and Moorish influences of the past to the more recent impact of global trade and colonization, Portuguese cuisine has been shaped by a wide range of cultural and historical factors.

One of the defining moments in the history of Portuguese cuisine was the Age of Discovery, when Portuguese explorers sailed the world in search of new trade routes and exotic ingredients. This period of exploration brought a wide range of new spices and ingredients to Portugal, including cinnamon, cloves, nutmeg, and pepper.

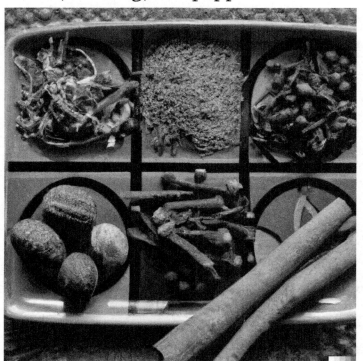

Another significant influence on Portuguese cuisine was the country's colonization of Brazil, which brought a variety of new ingredients to the country, including corn, beans, and various tropical fruits.

Today, Portuguese cuisine continues to evolve and adapt to changing tastes and influences, while still retaining its distinct culinary heritage and traditions.

Characteristics of Portuguese Cuisine

One of the defining characteristics of Portuguese cuisine is its focus on fresh, seasonal ingredients. From the seafood caught off the coast to the fruits and vegetables grown in the fertile valleys of the interior, Portuguese cuisine is centered around the natural bounty of the land and sea.

Another key characteristic of Portuguese cuisine is its use of bold flavors and spices. From the piri piri peppers used in chicken dishes to the garlic and onion found in many stews and soups, Portuguese cuisine is known for its rich and complex flavor profile.

Portuguese cuisine also places a strong emphasis on simplicity and comfort. Many traditional dishes are hearty and filling, designed to provide sustenance for the hardworking farmers and fishermen who make up much of the country's population.

Finally, Portuguese cuisine is characterized by its regional diversity. From the seafood-focused cuisine of the coast to the meat-heavy dishes of the interior, each region of Portugal has its own unique culinary traditions and specialties.

Key Ingredients in Portuguese Cooking

Several key ingredients are essential to the distinct flavor profile of Portuguese cuisine. Let's take a closer look at some of the most important ones:

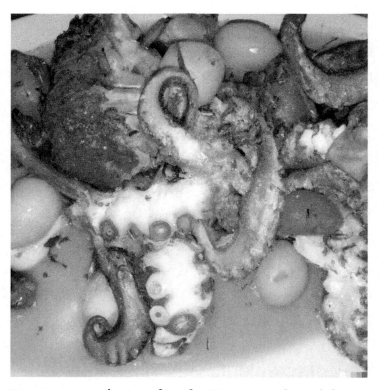

Portuguese' seafood Prepared with octopus

Seafood: Portugal's long coastline means that seafood is a central component of the country's cuisine.

From salt cod (bacalhau) to sardines, clams, and octopus, seafood is used in a wide variety of dishes, both simple and complex.

Olive Oil: Portugal is one of the largest producers of olive oil in the world, and this ingredient is a staple of Portuguese cooking. It's used to sauté vegetables, flavor stews and soups, and dress salads.

Garlic and Onion: These two ingredients are the foundation of many Portuguese dishes, particularly stews and soups. They add depth and complexity to dishes without overwhelming the other flavors.

Piri Piri Peppers: These small, fiery peppers are a key component of many Portuguese dishes, particularly chicken dishes. They add a spicy kick to the dish without overpowering the other flavors.

Rice: Rice is a staple of Portuguese cuisine, particularly in the form of arroz de marisco (seafood rice) and arroz de pato (duck rice). It's also used as a side dish to accompany stews and other main courses.

Wine: Portugal is known for its excellent wines, particularly port wine from the Douro Valley region. Wine is a central component of many Portuguese meals, and it's often paired with specific dishes to enhance the flavors.

Chouriço and other cured meats: Chouriço is a type of sausage that's commonly used in Portuguese cooking. It's made with pork and flavored with garlic and paprika, and it adds a rich, savory flavor to stews, soups, and other dishes.

Beans: Beans are a staple of Portuguese cuisine, particularly in the form of feijão frade (black-eyed peas) and feijão encarnado (red kidney beans). They're used in a wide range of dishes, from stews to salads.

Cabbage: Cabbage is a key ingredient in many Portuguese soups and stews, adding a subtle sweetness and depth of flavor to the dish.

Bread: Bread is an essential component of many Portuguese meals, particularly as an accompaniment to soups and stews. The country is known for its wide range of bread varieties, from crusty loaves to soft rolls.

These are just a few of the key ingredients that are essential to Portuguese cooking. By using fresh, high-quality ingredients and incorporating these traditional flavors, Portuguese chefs are able to create dishes that are both comforting and satisfying, while still showcasing the unique culinary heritage of the country.

Portuguese cuisine is a rich and diverse culinary tradition that's shaped by centuries of history, culture, and geography. From the fresh seafood of the coast to the hearty stews of the interior, Portuguese cuisine offers a wide range of flavors and textures that reflect the country's unique culinary heritage.

In this chapter, we've explored the history and characteristics of Portuguese cuisine, as well as some of the key ingredients that are essential to its distinct flavor profile. By using fresh, seasonal ingredients and incorporating bold flavors and spices, Portuguese chefs are able to create dishes that are both delicious and satisfying, while still staying true to the country's rich culinary traditions.

In the following chapters, we'll dive deeper into the different regions of Portugal and explore some of the country's most iconic dishes and wines. Whether you're a seasoned foodie or simply looking to explore new flavors and cuisines, we hope this guide will inspire you to discover the unique and delicious tastes of Portugal.

Chapter 2: A Culinary Tour of Portugal

Portugal is a country that's rich in culinary traditions, and each region has its own unique flavors and ingredients. In this chapter, we'll take you on a culinary tour of Portugal, exploring the distinctive dishes and wines of each region.

Lisbon and Surroundings

Lisbon is Portugal's capital and largest city, and it's home to a vibrant culinary scene that's steeped in tradition. One of the city's most iconic dishes is bacalhau, or salt cod, which is served in a wide range of preparations.

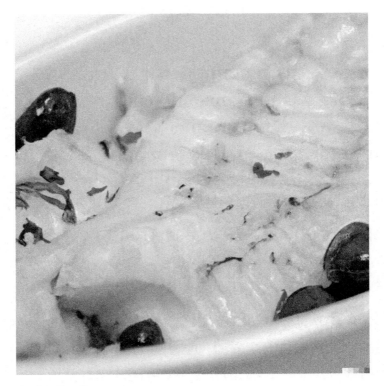

Salt Cod

Other popular dishes in Lisbon include cozido, a hearty stew made with a variety of meats and vegetables, and sardinhas assadas, grilled sardines that are a staple of Portuguese summertime cuisine.

Lisbon is also home to some of Portugal's best seafood restaurants, with a particular emphasis on dishes featuring shellfish like clams and prawns. The city's surrounding regions, like Cascais and Sintra, are known for their fresh seafood and also for their desserts, such as the famous pastéis de nata, or custard tarts.

Porto and the Douro Valley

Porto is Portugal's second-largest city and is famous for its production of port wine.

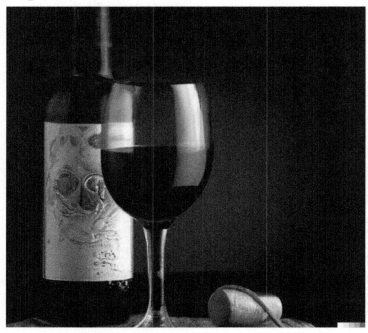

The Douro Valley, which surrounds the city, is a UNESCO World

Heritage site and is home to some of the world's most famous vineyards.

In addition to port wine, the region is also known for its rich, hearty cuisine. One of the most iconic dishes is cozido à portuguesa, a stew made with a variety of meats, vegetables, and beans. Another popular dish is tripeiro, a stew made with tripe and white beans that's said to have been invented by the city's tripe vendors.

Alentejo Region

The Alentejo region is located in the south-central part of Portugal and is known for its rustic, traditional cuisine. The region's most famous dish is migas, a hearty bread-based dish that's typically served with meat, vegetables, or fish.

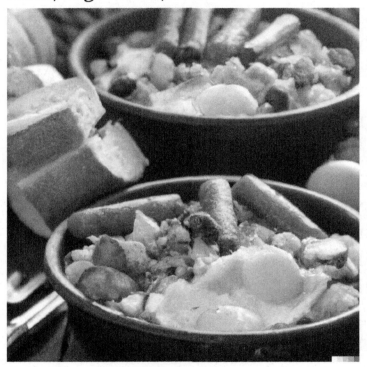

Migas

Other popular dishes include açorda, a soup made with bread and eggs, and ensopado de borrego, a lamb stew that's slow-cooked with herbs and spices.

The region is also known for its wines, particularly red wines made from grapes like Aragonês and Trincadeira.

Algarve Region

The Algarve region is located in the southernmost part of Portugal, and it's known for its fresh seafood and bright, bold flavors. Some of the region's most iconic dishes include cataplana, a seafood stew made with clams, shrimp, and chorizo, and sopa de peixe, a hearty fish soup that's served with crusty bread.

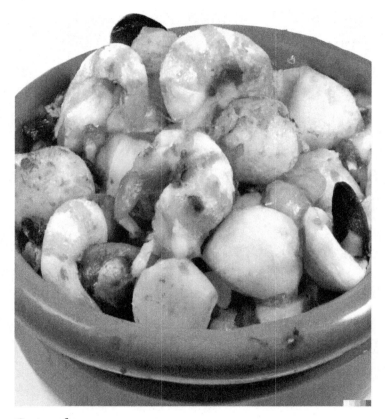

Cataplana

The region is also home to a variety of citrus fruits, which are often used in desserts like orange cake and fig and almond tart.

Madeira Island

Madeira is an island off the coast of Portugal, and it's famous for its rich, sweet fortified wines. The island's cuisine is also heavily influenced by its location in the Atlantic Ocean, with a focus on fresh seafood and tropical fruits.

One of the most iconic dishes of Madeira is espetada, a skewered meat dish that's marinated in garlic and bay leaves and grilled over an open flame.

Another popular dish is bolo do caco, a round flatbread that's typically served with garlic butter or grilled meat.

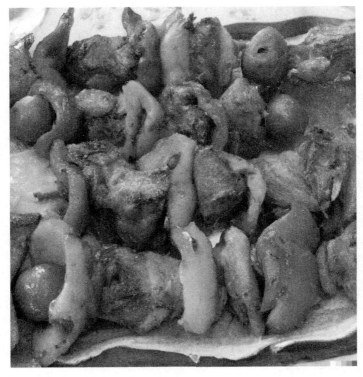

Espetada

Azores Island

The Azores Islands are a group of nine volcanic islands located in the Atlantic Ocean. The region is known for its dairy products, including cheese and butter, as well as its fresh seafood and hearty stews.

One of the most iconic dishes of the Azores is cozido das Furnas, a stew that's slow-cooked in volcanic steam vents. The stew typically includes a variety of meats, vegetables, and beans, and is served with bread or rice. Another popular dish is lapas, a type of limpet that's often grilled and served with garlic butter.

The Azores are also known for their wines, particularly the Ver

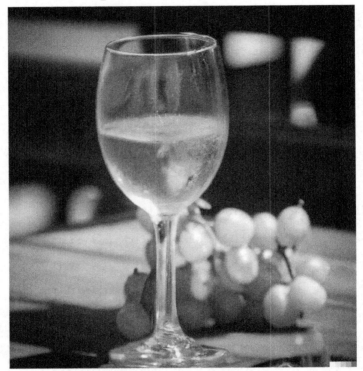

delho variety, which is a dry white wine with notes of tropical fruit and citrus.

Portugal's cuisine is a reflection of its long and storied history, as well as its unique geography and climate. From the hearty stews of the north to the fresh seafood of the south, each region has its own distinctive flavors and ingredients.

Whether you're a seasoned foodie or a casual traveler looking to experience something new, a culinary tour of Portugal is sure to be a feast for the senses. So why not grab a glass of port wine, dig into a plate of bacalhau, and explore the rich and vibrant culinary traditions of this beautiful country?

Chapter 3: Must-Try Portuguese Dishes

Bacalhau à Brás (Salt Cod with Potatoes and Eggs)

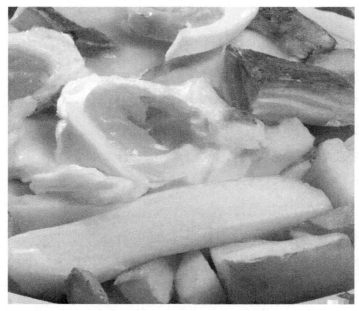

Bacalhau à Brás is one of the most iconic dishes in Portuguese cuisine.

Made with salt cod, potatoes, eggs, onions, and parsley, this dish is a classic example of Portuguese home-style cooking. The cod is soaked in water to remove the excess salt, then flaked and mixed with fried potatoes and onions. Finally, scrambled eggs are added to the mixture, and everything is seasoned with salt, pepper, and parsley. The result is a flavorful and satisfying dish that is a must-try for anyone visiting Portugal.

Cozido à Portuguesa (Portuguese Stew)

Cozido à Portuguesa is a hearty stew that is a staple in Portuguese cuisine. The dish is made with a variety of meats, such as beef, pork, chicken, and chouriço (a type of Portuguese sausage), along with a range of vegetables like carrots, turnips, and cabbage.

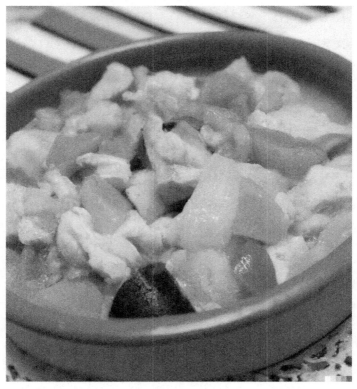

The stew is slowly cooked for hours, allowing the flavors to meld together and create a rich and satisfying dish. Cozido à Portuguesa is typically served with rice or potatoes and is a great option for a cold winter day.

Francesinha (Portuguese Sandwich)

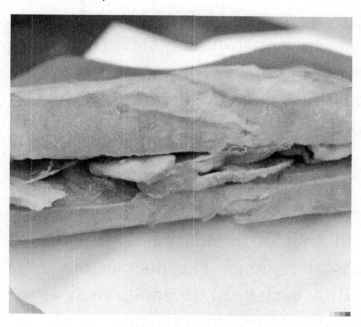

Francesinha is a unique sandwich that originated in Porto, Portugal. The sandwich is made with layers of bread, ham, linguiça (a type of Portuguese sausage), steak, and melted cheese, and is served in a spicy tomato-based sauce. The sandwich is then topped with a fried egg and served with a side of fries. The combination of flavors and textures makes Francesinha a must-try dish for anyone visiting Porto

Arroz de Marisco (Seafood Rice)

Arroz de Marisco is a seafood rice dish that is popular in Portugal's coastal regions. The dish is made with a variety of seafood, such as shrimp, clams, mussels, and squid, and is cooked with rice and vegetables like tomatoes, peppers, and onions.

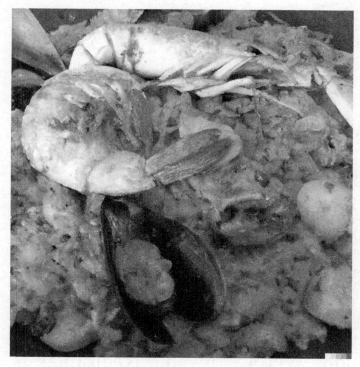

The dish is typically seasoned with garlic and parsley and is a great option for seafood lovers.

Caldo Verde (Green Soup)

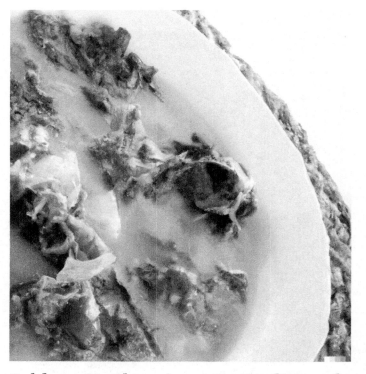

Caldo Verde is a traditional Portuguese soup that is made with potatoes, collard greens, and chouriço. The soup is typically seasoned with garlic and olive oil and is a great option for a cold winter day. The collard greens give the soup its distinct green color and add a unique flavor to the dish.

Pasteis de Nata (Portuguese Custard Tarts)

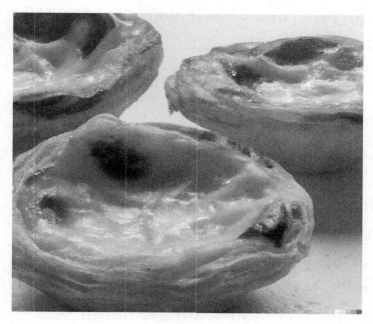

No guide to Portuguese cuisine would be complete without mentioning Pasteis de Nata. These custard tarts are a national treasure and are enjoyed by locals and tourists alike. The tarts are made with a flaky pastry shell and filled with a creamy egg custard. The tarts are typically served warm and are best enjoyed with a cup of Portuguese coffee.

Portuguese cuisine is a diverse and flavorful cuisine that is sure to satisfy even the most discerning food lovers. From seafood rice dishes to hearty stews and custard tarts, Portugal offers a range of must-try dishes that showcase the country's unique culinary heritage.

In this chapter, we highlighted some of the most iconic and popular dishes in Portuguese cuisine. Bacalhau à Brás, Cozido à Portuguesa, Francesinha, Arroz de Marisco, Caldo Verde, and Pasteis de Nata are all dishes that are loved by locals and visitors alike. Whether you're a seafood lover or a meat enthusiast, there is a Portuguese dish that is sure to delight your taste buds.

When visiting Portugal, we highly recommend trying these must-try dishes to get a true taste of the country's culinary culture. These dishes are not only delicious but also represent the history and traditions of Portugal's food culture.

In the next chapter, we will delve into the world of Portuguese wines and highlight some of the best wines that are produced in the country. Whether you're a wine connoisseur or a casual wine drinker, Portugal offers a range of wines that are sure to impress. So, let's raise a glass and explore the world of Portuguese wines.

Chapter 4: Wines of Portugal

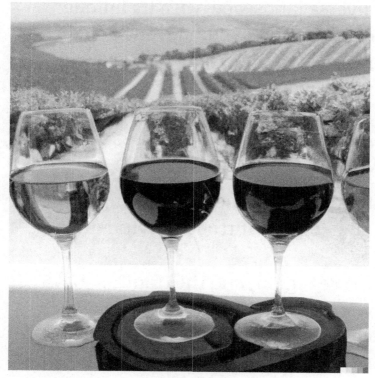

Portugal is a country with a long
history of winemaking. Wine has

been produced in the country for over 2,000 years, making Portugal one of the oldest wine-producing regions in the world. The country's diverse landscape, with its unique combination of climate and soil, has resulted in the production of a wide variety of high-quality wines.

A Brief History of Portuguese Wine

Winemaking in Portugal dates back to the time of the Roman Empire. The Romans introduced viticulture

to the region, and the tradition of winemaking has continued ever since. Over the centuries, Portuguese wine has been influenced by a variety of factors, including the country's maritime exploration, which led to the discovery of new grape varieties and winemaking techniques.

During the 20th century, Portugal faced challenges in its wine industry due to political and economic turmoil. However, in recent years, there has been a resurgence of interest in Portuguese wine, with the country's winemakers focusing on producing high-quality wines that showcase the unique character of Portugal's wine regions.

Portuguese Wine Regions

Portugal is divided into several wine regions, each with its own unique characteristics and styles of wine.

Some of the most well-known wine regions in Portugal include:

Douro Valley: Located in northern Portugal, the Douro Valley is known for producing some of the world's finest port wines. The region's steep terraced vineyards and hot, dry climate create ideal conditions for producing concentrated, flavorful wines.

Vinho Verde: Located in the northwest of Portugal, Vinho Verde is known for its light, crisp white wines. The region's cool, wet climate and granite soil create wines that are fresh, acidic, and aromatic.

Alentejo: Located in southern Portugal, Alentejo is known for its full-bodied red wines. The region's hot, dry climate and clay soil create wines that are rich, fruity, and spicy.

Dão: Located in central Portugal, the Dão region is known for producing elegant, complex red wines. The region's cool, mountainous climate and granite soil create wines that are balanced, structured, and age-worthy.

Grape Varieties in Portuguese Wine

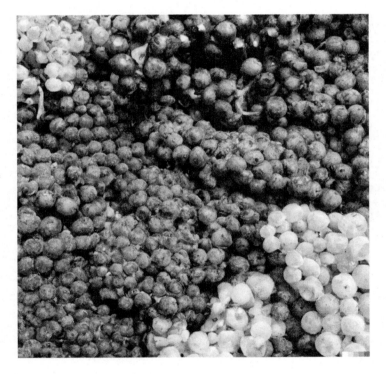

Portugal has a wide variety of indigenous grape varieties that are used to produce its wines. Some of the most common grape varieties in Portuguese wine include:

Touriga Nacional: A thick-skinned grape variety that is used to produce high-quality red wines, particularly port wines.

Alvarinho: A white grape variety that is used to produce Vinho Verde wines. It is known for its aromatic, floral, and citrusy flavors.

Aragonês: A red grape variety that is widely planted in Portugal. It is used to produce full-bodied red wines that are rich and spicy.

Baga: A red grape variety that is primarily grown in the Bairrada region of Portugal. It is used to produce full-bodied, tannic red wines that are known for their aging potential.

Must-Try Portuguese Wines

Portugal produces a wide variety of high-quality wines, ranging from light, crisp whites to full-bodied reds and sweet fortified wines. Some of the must-try Portuguese wines include:

Port: A fortified wine that is produced in the Douro Valley. Port wines are typically sweet and rich, with flavors of dried fruits, nuts, and spices.

Vinho Verde: A light, crisp white wine that is produced in the Vinho Verde region. Vinho Verde wines are known for their acidity, freshness, and aromatics.

Douro Red: A full-bodied red wine that is produced in the Douro Valley. Douro Reds are known for their deep, rich flavors of black fruit, chocolate, and spices.

Bairrada Red: A full-bodied red wine that is produced in the Bairrada region. Bairrada Reds are known for their firm tannins and flavors of dark fruit, tobacco, and earthy notes.

Dão Red: A complex red wine that is produced in the Dão region. Dão Reds are known for their elegance, with flavors of red fruit, herbs, and spices.

Madeira: A fortified wine that is produced on the island of Madeira. Madeira wines are known for their rich, complex flavors, with notes of caramel, honey, and nuts.

In addition to these must-try wines, Portugal also produces a range of other high-quality wines, including sparkling wines, rosés, and dessert wines.

Portugal's cuisine and wines are a reflection of the country's rich history and culture. From the seafood dishes of the coastal regions to the hearty stews of the interior, Portugal's cuisine offers a diverse range of flavors and textures. Similarly, Portugal's wine regions produce a wide variety of high-quality wines, each with its own unique character and style.

Whether you are a food lover or a wine enthusiast, exploring the flavors of Portugal is sure to be a memorable experience.

By trying some of the must-try dishes and wines outlined in this guide, you can get a taste of what makes Portugal's cuisine and wines so special. So, what are you waiting

for? Start planning your culinary
adventure to Portugal today!

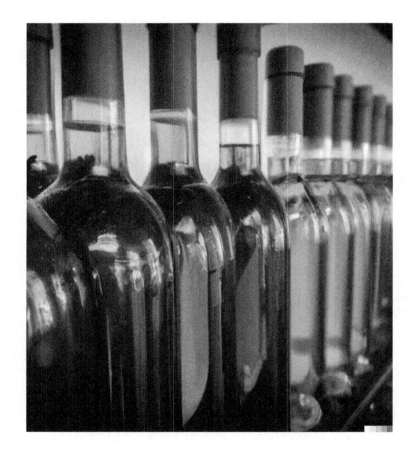

Chapter 5: Portuguese Culinary Phrases

If you're planning a trip to Portugal or simply want to explore Portuguese cuisine, it can be helpful to know some common culinary phrases and terminology.

In this chapter, we will provide a guide to useful Portuguese phrases for ordering food, common culinary terminology, and a pronunciation guide.

Useful Portuguese Phrases for Ordering Food

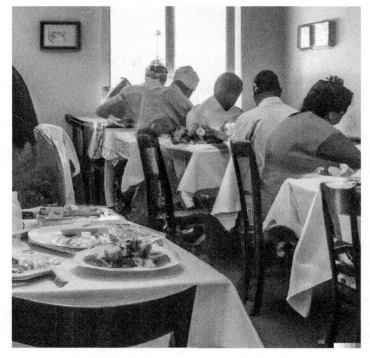

Here are some common Portuguese phrases that can be useful when ordering food at a restaurant or cafe:

O menu, por favor. (The menu, please.) – Use this phrase to ask for the menu at a restaurant or cafe.

Quero pedir agora. (I want to order now.) – Use this phrase to let the waiter know that you are ready to order.

Eu gostaria de... (I would like...) – Use this phrase to start your order.

O que você recomenda? (What do you recommend?) – Use this phrase to ask the waiter for their recommendation on what to order.

Tem alguma opção vegetariana?
(Do you have any vegetarian
options?) – Use this phrase to ask if
there are any vegetarian dishes on
the menu.

Por favor, sem... (Please, without...)
– Use this phrase to request that an
ingredient be removed from your
dish, such as "sem carne" (without
meat) or "sem queijo" (without
cheese).

Para beber, eu quero... (To drink, I
want...) – Use this phrase to order a
drink, such as "um copo de vinho
tinto" (a glass of red wine) or "uma
cerveja" (a beer).

A conta, por favor. (The bill, please.) – Use this phrase to ask for the bill at the end of your meal.

Common Portuguese Culinary Terminology

Here are some common culinary terms that you might come across when exploring Portuguese cuisine:

Bacalhau – Salt cod, a staple ingredient in Portuguese cuisine.

Chouriço – A type of sausage made with pork and spices.

Frango – Chicken.

Gambas – Prawns.

Leitão - Suckling pig, a popular dish in central Portugal.

Polvo - Octopus, often served grilled or in a stew.

Queijo - Cheese, with varieties such as queijo da serra and queijo fresco.

Sopa - Soup, with popular varieties including caldo verde and sopa de tomate.

Pronunciation Guide

Portuguese pronunciation can be tricky for non-native speakers, but here are some tips to help you get started:

The letter "c" is pronounced like "s" before "e" and "i" (e.g. "cerveja" is pronounced "ser-vey-ja").

The letter "s" is pronounced like "sh" before "i" (e.g. "sopa" is pronounced "sho-pa").

The letter "j" is pronounced like the "s" in "pleasure" (e.g. "bacalhau" is pronounced "ba-kal-yow").

The letter "r" is pronounced like a rolled "r" (e.g. "frango" is pronounced "frran-go").

The letter "u" is often silent in Portuguese (e.g. "queijo" is pronounced "kay-zho").

Conclusion

Exploring Portuguese cuisine is a delightful experience that can be made even more enjoyable by knowing some common culinary phrases and terminology.

By using the phrases provided in this chapter, you can confidently order food at a restaurant or cafe, and by familiarizing yourself with common culinary terminology, you can better understand the dishes you are trying.

Remember to also practice your Portuguese pronunciation to make your dining experience even more authentic.

I hope this guide has been helpful in your culinary journey through Portugal. Bom apetite! (Enjoy your meal!)

Tips for Enjoying Portuguese Cuisine to the Fullest

Here are some tips for enjoying Portuguese cuisine to the fullest:

Try the seafood: Portugal is known for its delicious seafood dishes, such as grilled sardines, octopus, and bacalhau (salt cod). Be sure to try these dishes when you have the chance.

Experiment with the cheese: Portugal has a wide variety of delicious cheeses, such as queijo da

serra, queijo fresco, and azeitão.
Pair them with local wines or fruits
for an even better experience.

Order a Francesinha: This is a
popular sandwich in Porto that is
made with bread, ham, sausage,
and steak, topped with melted
cheese and a tomato-based sauce.
It's a hearty and delicious meal that
you shouldn't miss.

Don't forget the wine: Portugal has
a long history of winemaking, and
there are many excellent wines to
try. Some popular varieties include
port wine, vinho verde, and red
wines from the Douro region.

Try the traditional sweets: Portugal has many traditional sweets, such as pastel de nata (custard tarts), arroz doce (rice pudding), and queijadas (sweet cheese pastries). Be sure to save room for dessert!

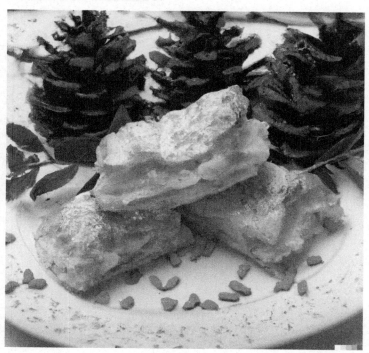

Printed in Great Britain
by Amazon

24758382R00040